LOVING MY WIFE BACK TO HEALTH

LOVING MY WIFE BACK TO HEALTH

TOM WILLIAMS

SWORD of the LORD
PUBLISHERS
P. O. BOX 1099, MURFREESBORO, TN 37133

TWICE GIVEN FOR GOD'S GLORY
Copyright 1981 by Tom Williams

LOVING MY WIFE BACK TO HEALTH
Revised edition: 1992

Copyright 1992 by Tom Williams

ISBN-0-87398-523-0

If your local bookstore does not have this book, additional
copies at $4.95 each (plus shipping and handling) may be
obtained from Sword of the Lord Publishers, or directly
from Dr. Williams' office:

> Tom Williams Ministries
> HCR 66; Box 44-D
> West Plains, MO 65775
> Telephone: 417/257-7797

Printed and Bound in the United States of America

Dedication

Dedicated to my four wonderful children and their spouses.

Thank you for all the blessing, encouragement and strength you have been to me during these many years.

Contents

Acknowledgments

This page cannot contain all the names of folks who have been such a vital part of our lives through my wife's traumatic illness and our family's trials, but I have done my best to include them in these pages.

In addition, I want to express my sincere appreciation to my secretary, Sue Cawthron, for the many hours she spent typing, editing and verifying information for this book, which was originally published under the title, *Twice Given for God's Glory.*

I'm grateful to Dr. James Dobson for broadcasting the story of our testimony several times on his "Focus on the Family" radio program, using the title, "Loving My Wife Back to Health." Folks throughout the country have used his title many times in referring to our story.

Since we were re-editing the original book, we decided to change the title to *Loving My Wife Back to Health.* I trust that it will be a rich blessing to your heart as you read it.

"When Jesus heard that, he said, This sickness is not unto death, but for the glory of God, that the Son of God might be glorified thereby."—John 11:4.

CHAPTER 1

Teenage Bride

Pamela Marie James came into my life in the summer of 1958, following the death of my first wife Wanda. Pam was just a young girl, between her junior and senior years of high school, when I met her. Even at that young age, she already was serving the Lord.

I had gone to visit my first wife's brother, Rev. E. B. Claud, who was working with the American Sunday School Union in establishing Sunday schools in out-of-the-way places. I didn't know that Pam was living with his family for the summer to help in his work.

When my two-year-old son Tim and I walked into E. B.'s home that day, there stood a beautiful young girl. The Lord spoke to my heart and told me she was the girl He wanted me to marry. I immediately said, "But, Father, she is so young."

He replied, "Tom, if you don't want the one I have for you, then you may find your own."

Needless to say, without any further argument, I set out to win her heart.

It didn't take long that afternoon to learn that Pam was only sixteen years old. She was from Hemet, California, a small town about 100 miles east of Los Angeles. Pam came from a fine Christian home and was the oldest of three girls.

She and her family attended the First Baptist Church of Hemet.

I told her that weekend what the Lord had told me about her. She immediately replied, "I don't understand all that is happening; but when you walked in the door today and your eyes met mine, I knew you were the man I was going to marry."

God led in our courtship, and we began to date in September. We were married the following year on July 10. God gave Pam to me in answer to my prayer for a mother for Tim and a wife for myself. . . someone who would love me and stand by my side. . . someone to help heal my broken heart and fill the emptiness in our lives. And this was our idea in dating. I realized that was a tremendous responsibility for such a young woman, but Pam did an excellent job.

As Tim and I both have testified many times, Pam was sent from God to meet our needs. It was for God's glory that He gave her to us because He knew that both Tim and I would one day be in the ministry and would need someone very special.

Some of you no doubt are wondering, *You mean she was only seventeen years of age when you married her?* Yes, and we married with the full approval and blessings of her dad and mother.

Although I don't believe everyone should marry at a young age, some of the sweetest couples I know are those who married while they were young.

Some folks are as mature at seventeen as others are at twenty-two or twenty-three. Pam was one of those young ladies. She stepped right into the role of wife and mother, picked up the reins of motherhood and did a wonderful job with Tim. She also was a fantastic wife—just what the Great Physician ordered to soothe the sorrows of my heart, as well as to build a man whom God would use all across America and around much of the world.

Those early years of our marriage were wonderful days for

us. Since Pam was only thirteen years older than Tim, we faced many amusing situations.

When we took Tim to get his polio vaccination, the lady at the desk asked our ages. I told her I was twenty-six and Pam was nineteen. With a shocked look on her face, the lady looked up at me and asked, "How old is the boy?"

Very calmly I replied, "Six."

When we walked out of her office, she was still sitting there in a daze, staring at us. We could hardly wait to get out of sight so we could have a good laugh!

At another time we were at a wedding in Los Angeles, where I was to take part in the ceremony. Just before the wedding, Pam and another woman were talking. The lady was telling Pam how much work was involved in having a child in the second grade, and she mentioned that, with so much to do, she was almost late.

Pam was twenty at the time, but she looked more like seventeen. When she told the lady that she certainly could sympathize with her, being a mother of two herself and one of them a second grader, the woman practically gasped out loud.

When Pam was only nineteen, God called me to be a full-time evangelist. She was left at home with two children and all the responsibilities that go along with running a home. It soon became apparent just how mature Pam really was. I was gone for six to eight weeks at a time in those early days, but she never complained.

Let me say that I have since learned how wrong I was to be gone from home for such long periods of time and to put so much pressure on her, the children and our marriage.

Like many other evangelists, I used the argument that I had to be gone that much in order to make it financially. But the Lord taught me an important lesson: God is not the author of confusion. He does not give a man a family, then ask him to neglect his responsibilities as husband and father.

God blessed our marriage by giving Pam and me three

children in addition to Tim. Pam had turned eighteen in February before our first child, Phyllis Ann, was born on July 23, 1960. Tim was elated. When I told him that Mommy and the baby would be coming home in a couple of days, he asked, "Can sister and I play together in the backyard?"

Had I known then that I would be away from home when our next two children were newborn, I would have cherished those days so much more.

When Phyllis was almost three years old, Pam gave birth to our second son, Thomas Paul, on May 4, 1963, at 5:30 a.m. I had to leave at 8:00 a.m.—just two and one-half hours later—for four weeks of meetings. (As I think back to those times, I am amazed at Pam's patience and understanding with me. I am sure that those thoughts of her desire to be what I needed and to do nothing that would hinder the ministry are what drove me on in the long days of the trial of her illness years later.)

Tim was almost twelve, Phyllis was crowding seven, and Paul was just two months away from being four when our little girl, Penny Ruth, was born on March 10, 1967, at 9:30 p.m. I was in a meeting when Pam went into labor, and I didn't get to the hospital until about thirty minutes after Penny was born.

Pam had prayed for a little girl that would have her features—brunette hair, brown eyes, an olive complexion— and God answered her prayers. Many times down through the years, various people have told our daughter, "Penny, you look just like your mother."

For fifteen years I traveled alone in the work of evangelism. As I said, Pam never complained, and she did a super job of rearing the children and keeping things going at home. Our pastor, Dr. Ed Rodda of the First Baptist Church of Hemet, California, told me, "Tom, you married not only one of the prettiest girls in the world, but also one of the finest." I agreed wholeheartedly.

While I laid the foundation years of my ministry, Pam did

what few women would do or could do: she reared the children with strict discipline mingled with precious love so that today every one of them is saved and living for the Lord. Truly it was for God's glory that He gave Pam to me.

CHAPTER 2

The Beginning of the Almost End

It is the Lord's giving Pam to me the second time that will occupy most of this book. It will take us from the beginning of our tour of Israel all the way down through the Valley of the Shadow of Death.

When Dr. Tom Berry of Elkton, Maryland, asked me to co-host a tour to the Bible lands, I had mixed emotions. For years folks had asked me to go to Israel, but I had always put off the trip, saying I didn't want to see all the commercialism.

As I prayed and talked to various people about the trip, I became excited about going.

We received the brochures and began making contacts. Soon we had a group from many different states—Washington, Ohio, Alabama, Florida, Colorado, Virginia, Michigan, Indiana, New York and North Carolina. We were thankful that five of the team members of the Tom Williams Ministries would be going: Bud and Sherry Grinstead, our son Tim, along with Pam and me.

We were scheduled to meet at John F. Kennedy Airport in New York on February 26, 1978. My family and I drove up from North Carolina, where we had just finished a meeting with Pastor D. O. Lingafelt and the people of Friendship Baptist Church. We stopped in Springfield, Virginia, a suburb of Washington, D.C., to leave our three youngest children with some of our very precious friends, Mr. and Mrs. Warren Hosaflook. We left our motor home at the Rose Hill Baptist Church, not far from where the children would be staying. Then Tim, Pam and I flew on up to New York.

The people in our tour group began to arrive from all over the country, and excitement mounted as departure time drew near. Soon everyone was accounted for, visas and passports were in order, and we were ushered onto our 747 jet, along with Dr. Tom Berry and his group, making a total of fifty-six people in the two groups.

The jet was soon in the air, and we were on our way to our first destination—Amsterdam. We arrived there in the morning and were told that we would have an unexpected layover of about four hours. Dr. Berry and I chartered some buses and took our group on a tour of Amsterdam, a beautiful city with its canals, Dutch windmills and flowers.

As we finished our tour and arrived back at the airport, it was time for the plane to leave for our second destination—Amman, Jordan.

Landing in Amman was a different kind of experience, to say the least. Guards with automatic weapons surrounded us as we deplaned and escorted us into Customs, maintaining very tight security.

After they finished checking through our luggage, our guide ushered us outside. It was comical to watch the Jordanian tour guides as they yelled back and forth at each other and to the drivers, trying to make sure the tourists got to their correct buses. Finally we boarded our tour bus and were taken to our hotel for a night of much-needed sleep.

The next day we went down to Petra, the rose-red rock city of the dead, and to Nebo, the mountain where Moses was taken by God. Our guide, Sabri, kept us entertained with his jokes and good sense of humor.

We had a thrilling time the next day as we approached the banks of the Jordan River to leave the country of Jordan and go over into Israel, crossing at the Allenby Bridge. An interesting experience awaited us there, too.

Because of the tense military situation in the Middle East, heavily armed Jordanian soldiers guarded one side of the river while Jewish soldiers guarded the Israeli side—ready to fire at any moment should enemy soldiers try to cross over.

On the Israeli side, we started through Jewish Customs. They were much stricter than in any of the other countries we had visited. The ladies were searched by women Customs officials, and the men searched by men. They looked through everyone's luggage, searching for possible hidden weapons or bombs that anyone might be bringing into the country. They also X-rayed the heels of some of the people's shoes and cut the lining out of some of the suitcases because they were the type that sometimes are used to smuggle things into the country. We had to flash our cameras to let the officials know we were not hiding explosives inside the cameras.

After everyone got through Israeli Customs, we met our guide, a Jewish man named Malcolm. Although he was not saved, Malcolm had a tremendous knowledge of the Word of God, and he carried the Bible everywhere he went.

Malcolm showed us the city of Jericho, including a sycamore tree similar to the one Zacchaeus climbed so that he could see Jesus, the spring of water which Elisha purified after Elijah was taken by God on the other side of Jordan, and the ruins of the walls which fell when Joshua and the Israelites marched around the city. We also saw the Mount of Temptation and the wilderness where the Lord Jesus stayed for forty days and nights.

Then we made our way up the Jericho Road toward Jerusalem, stopping at the halfway point where the Good Samaritan helped the man who had been beaten and left for dead (Luke 10:30-35).

I'll never forget our first glimpse of Jerusalem. My heart skipped a beat at the breathtaking view of the city where our Lord Jesus spent so much of His time when He was on earth, the city where so many Bible events took place.

We were a little disappointed when Malcolm told us that we would be going to Bethlehem before we toured Jerusalem. But I'm glad now that we did, as we were able to see Jesus' birthplace first and then see the city where He carried on much of His ministry and was later crucified.

What a thrill to stand in the traditional cave of His birth and realize that the Son of God, incarnate in human flesh years ago, had lain there! An overwhelming sense of joy flooded our souls as we were reminded once again that our Saviour came from the glories of Heaven to a place of lowly birth to make a way for sinners like us to be accepted by Almighty God!

In Jerusalem we visited Calvary, the empty tomb, the Mount of Olives, the Garden of Gethsemane and the Dome of the Rock, which was built on the Temple Mount (where Abraham had bound Isaac, where David had bought the threshing floor from Ornan, and where Solomon had constructed the Temple). We also toured the narrow streets and marketplaces of the old city of Jerusalem. How interesting to walk on the streets where the Lord Jesus walked, taught and healed people!

From Jerusalem we journeyed north to the Sea of Galilee, stopping en route at Megiddo (also called "the Valley of Armageddon"), a 75-mile stretch of land where the Battle of Armageddon, the last battle of the world, will be fought. We saw the ruins of Solomon's stables and the ingenious way Solomon stored the grain and brought it up through a huge chasm. He very cleverly had designed the storage area with steps leading to a vast water supply underneath the mountain.

Then we went to the city of Nazareth in Galilee, where the Lord Jesus lived as a child, a teenager and part of His adult life.

In Cana, the city where Jesus performed His first miracle,

we visited a synagogue similar to the one where Jesus had taught. We crossed the Sea of Galilee and saw where the two thousand pigs had run off the cliff after the demons from the Gadarene demoniac had entered into the swine (Mark 5:1-13). What a thrill to be at the sea where Jesus had walked on the water and where Peter, John, Andrew and James had fished!

Right there on the Sea of Galilee we stopped the boat and had a preaching service. We also had services at Jacob's Well, at the ruins of the synagogue in Capernaum, and in many other places.

After having spent the night in a hotel along the seashore in Galilee, we stood on the shore the next morning and listened to Bud Grinstead sing "The Stranger of Galilee." That moving experience brought tears to many eyes as we were reminded again of our precious Saviour and His ministry on earth.

Some of the folks in our group wanted to be baptized in the Jordan River, so we stopped and had a baptismal service on our way back to Jerusalem.

Those were momentous times as we saw for the first time in our lives some of the things about which we had read and studied for years.

The next morning was the morning of Mrs. Williams' illness. When we got up, she had no visible symptoms of illness. We traveled down to the Dead Sea and passed Engedi, the area where David had hidden from Saul in a stronghold near the Dead Sea (I Sam. 23:27-29).

We were enthralled with the Dead Sea, a body of water which typifies many Christians. An abundance of wealth and life flows into the sea, but there is no outlet. Just as the Dead Sea contains a great treasure of minerals and other things, the Christian contains a great wealth of spiritual truth gained through the studying and preaching of the Word. But if there is no outlet for that life, it will dry up.

Leaving the Dead Sea that morning, we traveled to

Masada, the mountain where 900 Jewish zealots had taken their own lives many centuries earlier rather than let the Romans massacre them.

Even when we stepped inside the large aerial tram to go to the top of Masada, Pam seemingly was feeling all right. But just before we reached the top, she began to shake almost uncontrollably. Some of the people in our group loaned her their coats, but we were not able to stop the shaking. This was the beginning of the almost end, for Pam would step very close to the doors of death.

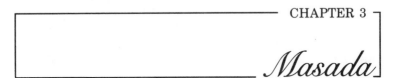

CHAPTER 3

Masada

Little did we know, as we topped the mountain where hundreds of Jews had ended their lives many centuries earlier, that Pam would begin a battle that would almost end her life. We didn't know that germs carrying bacterial meningitis had been hiding in her body and incubating for a period of ten to twelve days.

While the others toured Masada, Sherry Grinstead and Christy Candlish (a lady from Indiana who was on the tour with us) helped me with Pam. But no matter how many coats we put around her, we were not able to get her warm or make her comfortable.

After the others finished their tour of Masada, we helped Pam down the back side of the mountain. By that time she was having intense pain in her lower back. It grieved me that we were not able to make it easier for her.

There was only one way to get to the top of the mountain—on the large aerial tram. The only way off the mountain was to walk about a mile down a steep, winding trail on the other side. Even if we could have taken the tram back down, we would not have been able to go back to our bus and get help. After our driver had let us off at the base of Masada, he had left to drive several miles to the other side of the mountain, where he would be waiting to continue our tour after we got off the mountain.

We finally got Pam to the tour bus, and she was able to lie down in the back seat. The driver took us to the little town of Arad, Israel, and Malcolm arranged for an ambulance to take Pam to a hospital in Beersheba, about seventy miles away. The driver was very helpful to Tim and me as we tried to make Pam comfortable.

Trying to communicate with the hospital staff was a new experience for me, as many of them did not speak or understand English. Finally a Jewish nurse from America approached and, in fluent English, asked if she could help. We were so grateful for her. Later the Lord gave us an opportunity to witness to her.

The doctors in Beersheba examined Pam and ran a number of tests, trying to determine the cause of her illness.

Malcolm had taken the rest of our group sightseeing while Pam, Tim and I went on to the hospital. Later that day, they were anxious to know what was happening with Pam, so Malcolm asked the driver to go by the hospital. Malcolm found us and asked about Pam before continuing the tour. Since there was nothing we could do but pray and wait, I insisted that Tim rejoin the group and finish the tour.

Pam and I stayed at the hospital for about seven hours. After further X-rays and tests, the doctors kindly told me they had not been able to locate the source of Pam's pain and that she had developed a fever. They had thought that perhaps she had a kidney infection, but the tests showed very little infection there. Their advice was to get Pam back to the States as soon as possible and to get medical care in America.

We asked the Jewish nurse to call a taxicab and explain to the driver that we wanted to go to the hotel in Tel Aviv, about a hundred miles away, where our group would spend the night. I sat in the back seat so Pam could rest her head on my lap. She was very sick.

We finally arrived at the hotel, and Christy Candlish stayed up most of the night helping me with Pam. By this time we thought Pam had some kind of flu, but we had no idea that her situation was as serious as it really was.

The next morning our guide was very kind to talk to Customs officials, and Pam and I were able to quickly get through Customs and onto the plane. The Lord worked it out so graciously, as He always does. There was only one empty seat on the flight from Tel Aviv to Amsterdam, and they left that seat by us so Pam would have room to lie down with her head on my lap. By that time, the disease must have had a drugging effect on Pam, because all she wanted to do was sleep, for which we were thankful. We changed planes in Amsterdam, and she was able to sleep again.

We changed planes again at John F. Kennedy Airport in New York; and Tim, Pam and I flew on to Washington, D.C.

When the Hosaflooks met us at the airport, they were saddened to hear that Pam was ill. They took us to our motor home, and I asked Pam if she wanted to go to the hospital. Still coherent at the time, she replied, "No, I think I'll be all right if I can just get in bed, be still and quit flying."

Deciding to wait until morning to get the children, I put Pam to bed. She slept pretty well for about an hour, then woke up sicker than before.

I called the assistant pastor of the church where our motor home was parked, and he took us to the hospital where the pastor met us. When we admitted Pam to the Alexandria Hospital, little did we know how long she would stay and what a battle we would undergo. The doctor examined her and said that she was run down and dehydrated. He had the nurse begin intravenous feeding immediately. Not long afterward, the doctor came out and told me that the intravenous feeding had caused her electrolytes to pick up and there was a general improvement in her condition.

We had checked Pam into the hospital around 11:00 p.m. About 3:00 a.m., the nurse came to the waiting room and told me the doctor wanted to see me. As I walked in the room, the doctor asked, "Mr. Williams, did your wife learn some strange words in Israel?"

"No, not that I know of. Why?"

"She's talking very funny."

"Let me talk to her."

I went in and said, "Honey, I love you."

Pam replied, "I love you, too."

I turned to the doctor and said, "She's talking all right; she told me she loves me."

"Ask where she hurts."

Every time I asked Pam where she hurt, she said some strange words. . .words that meant nothing. I became very concerned when I realized that Pam's illness was affecting her mental capacity. I didn't know if Satan was trying to overpower her mind in this weakened condition, or just what was taking place; but we began to pray and plead the blood of Christ over her mind, her life and her body.

By that time the pain in her back was so excruciating that she could hardly stand it; she was kicking the steel frame of the bed with her bare feet.

I became impatient and asked the doctor to give her something to ease the pain, as she was hurting so terribly. The doctor explained that he could not give her any medication, as it was the pain that would help them determine what was causing the problem. At the time, I must admit I didn't have much patience with that theory, but afterwards I saw the validity of it.

Because of Pam's illness and the stress of the trip, I was extremely weary and didn't know what to do. I felt so helpless. I called our doctor in Denver (where we were living at that time) and told him the situation. Being so far away, there was nothing he could do, but he told me to keep him posted on what was happening.

Since the doctors at Alexandria Hospital had not been able to determine the cause of Pam's illness. . .and since she had been using strange words, her doctor suggested that a psychiatrist examine her. They thought Pam's problem was mental.

I tried to reason with them that it was the physical illness that somehow had caused the problem with her mind, and not the other way around. But her doctor refused to proceed any further unless I allowed him to call in a psychiatrist. It was either that, or Pam would have to leave.

I told him, "You know I can't take her out of the hospital; she is too ill to travel."

I considered moving her to Denver. I even called a friend (whom we will say more about later) and asked about using his private jet. That didn't work out, and I'm glad now that it didn't. Pam probably would have died on the way to Denver.

Not feeling I had any choice, I told the doctor, "All right, you can call a psychiatrist, but you cannot put my wife in a mental ward."

The doctor assured me that Pam would not be committed to a mental ward without my permission.

The psychiatrist was just a young man, about twenty-seven or twenty-eight years old, but he really was sent from God. He walked over to Pam's bed, talked to her for a couple of minutes, and asked her some questions. In the best way she could, Pam answered with her eyes and by nodding her head.

The psychiatrist turned and faced the medical doctors, giving his recommendation, "Whatever is wrong with this woman, it is *not* mental. You had better do something fast!"

At that point a Chinese doctor, an internal specialist named Dr. Shih, approached and told me he would take Pam's case. He asked me to sign for Pam to have a lower lumbar puncture immediately. Afterward Dr. Shih came out and said, "Rev. Williams, I never try to hide anything from my patients or their relatives. Your wife has the most severe case of bacterial meningitis that I have ever seen. She will probably be dead in twenty-four hours or less."

He continued, "I don't know how much you know about

medical things, but the spinal fluid is supposed to be about as clear as tap water. Your wife's spinal fluid has the consistency of buttermilk."

I didn't know what all that meant, but I asked if there was anything he could do for her. Dr. Shih explained that Pam had the meningococcal variety of meningitis, which will sometimes respond to penicillin. He said they could administer twenty-four million units of penicillin immediately, but that he really didn't think it would help. By this time Pam had lapsed into a coma after having convulsions and a grand mal seizure.

About three hours after Dr. Shih gave her the penicillin, he came to me again: "We must administer another twenty-four million units."

And for the next fourteen days, Pam received one million units of penicillin each hour, totaling just short of 350 million units. Since she had not awakened from the coma after fourteen days, the doctors were convinced at that point that she had no more than two days to live.

At Dr. Shih's request, three infectious-disease specialists had joined him in working on Pam's case. I already appreciated Dr. Shih's diligence and concern, and I felt especially blessed by God when I learned that there were only a small number of such specialists in America and that three of them were working with Pam.

When they discovered that Pam had bacterial meningitis, they quickly prescribed some medicine for Tim and me, as well as for the other children, in case we had the germ in our body. The doctors also advised me to notify all of the people who had been with us on the tour so they could have their local physicians prescribe medicine for them.

When I first learned the seriousness of Pam's condition, I called Dr. Ed Nelson, our pastor in Denver, Colorado, and told him. He alerted the church folks, and the ladies in the prayer chain began to call one another, joining their hearts in earnest prayer.

I called Dr. Bob Jones III at Bob Jones University in Greenville, South Carolina, and asked him to pray. He said, "Tom, you couldn't have called at a better time. This is a day of prayer at Bob Jones University."

At the chapel service he alerted the student body of Pam's illness. The faculty and thousands of students began to pray.

I also called Hyles-Anderson College in Indiana, and they began praying for Pam.

Dr. Lee Roberson and the students at Tennessee Temple Schools in Chattanooga began to pray. Christian day schools, colleges, churches and individuals all around the world united in prayer for my dear wife. Within just a few hours, tens of thousands of people were praying.

Eighteen years of evangelism began to pay dividends in a way I never dreamed.

CHAPTER 4

The Long Vigil

While Pam was in the Intensive Care Unit of Alexandria Hospital, many wires ran to her body from the various support machines. Since she was in a coma, we could not tell whether or not she knew we were there. But we continued to talk to her and pray for her just as though she could hear us.

The doctors had said that Pam probably wouldn't live more than twenty-four hours, so I knew I had to tell the children. I shall never forget the way they responded. Naturally, there were lots of tears, but they very sweetly accepted her illness as from the Lord.

We knelt along the couch at the home of the Hosaflooks, and each of the children prayed. Tim's birth mother had died when he was only two years old; now he faced the reality that his second mother might die. With tears cascading down his face, Tim prayed sincerely, "Lord, if You need Mother more than I do, I understand. I'll still serve You, and I'll still preach for You."

One by one the children committed their mother to the Lord. They told Him that, if He wanted her in Heaven, we would somehow make it without her.

Afterward I took the children to the hospital to see Pam. Although the younger ones were not allowed to stay very long, Tim and I stayed day and night for three or four days, leaving just long enough to shower, shave and change clothes.

As you can imagine, the first twenty-four hours passed very slowly. At the end of that time, Pam was still fighting the battle of life. The doctor told me, "Your wife made it through the first twenty-four hours. However, the next seventy-two are very critical. If she survives that long, she *may* have a chance."

So we started the long vigil of seventy-two additional hours. In the waiting room was a door leading to the hallway of the Intensive Care Unit. Each time it opened, my heart seemed to skip a beat, for that was the door the doctors used when they had to tell family members that a loved one had died.

Fifteen people died while we were waiting to see whether or not Pam would live, but I'm so grateful that the message never came through that door for the Williams family to start funeral arrangements.

Many times as I walked down the hall to the Intensive Care Unit, I prayed, "Lord, give Pam mercy and the children and me grace."

And again and again He did exactly that. One night as I was praying for Pam, the Lord reminded me of a verse of Scripture in Proverbs, which says the Word of God is "health to thy navel, and marrow to thy bones" (3:8).

Greatly encouraged, I got a cassette player and some cassette tapes of the Scriptures and took them to Pam's room. I told the nurses that I believed the Word of God is a healer and that I wanted Pam to hear the Scriptures. I put the earphone into Pam's ear and turned on the tape player. I asked the nurses to keep the tapes going twenty-four hours a day. I still didn't know if Pam could hear; but if she could, I wanted her to hear the Word of God constantly.

One of the doctors, a Jewish man named Dr. Goldberg, noticed the earphone in Pam's ear and asked, "What in the world is going on here?"

The nurse explained, "As you know, Rev. Williams is very

religious, and he said that the Bible says in the book of Proverbs that God's Word is health to the navel and strength to the bones. He knew that Mrs. Williams needed all the strength and help she could get."

Dr. Goldberg replied, "If the Old Testament says that, then it's true." And he wrote a medical prescription for the tape recording of the Word of God to be kept playing in Mrs. Williams' ear twenty-four hours a day!

We not only got a little chuckle out of that, but our family was blessed because God had worked in his heart to allow the playing of the tapes instead of asking us to remove them from her room.

We also were amused at the response of some of the nurses. Sometimes when we walked into Pam's room, one of the nurses would have the earphone plugged into *her* ear, listening to the tape. We were thankful that the Word of God was getting into other hearts also.

It was during this long vigil that one of the nurses came out of the Intensive Care Unit one day and said, "Mr. Williams, some of the nurses wanted me to ask you what is different about Mrs. Williams."

"What do you mean?"

"There is a radiance that comes from her that we have not seen in other patients."

I told her, "It's because she is full of God."

When Pam was transferred from Intensive Care to Acute Care a few days later, the nurses there asked me the same thing.

Before her illness, Pam had memorized many chapters of the Bible. She was a very godly woman and had a deep desire to please the Lord. She literally radiated the glory of God. It was so wonderful to see how God was still using Pam for His glory, even though she was in a coma and could not communicate.

Dr. Shih, the Chinese doctor who was treating Pam, came by the waiting room once or twice a day to give me a report on how he felt Pam was doing. Occasionally the nurses told me they thought they had seen some improvement in Pam's condition—her heartbeat seemed stronger, or her breathing seemed more even. But Dr. Shih told me very frankly, "When your wife sits up in bed and says, 'You are my husband,' then I will say, 'Your wife is better and is going to live.' "

Dr. Shih really did not think there was any hope for her.

Pam lived through the ninety-six-hour period and remained in the Intensive Care Unit for ten more days. The three infectious disease specialists checked her every day, pooling their medical knowledge in an effort to get some response from Pam; but there was no response.

At the end of the fourteen-day period they told me that Pam could not live; and that if by some miracle she were to survive, she would be a "vegetable." She would never recognize us, never know anything, never have any control over her system.

Immediately a struggle began in my mind to continue to believe that God was going to heal her. Was this it? Was Pam going to die? Praise the Lord, He helped me maintain faith.

Since the Intensive Care Unit was so terribly expensive, the doctors decided to move Pam to the Acute Care Unit. They said, "We can't do any more for her in Intensive Care than they can do there."

Of course, I knew they were really telling me there was no hope—that they were moving her down there to die.

Let me say that I certainly appreciated everything the doctors and nurses did. They were all very kind and took personal interest in our situation. When the doctors told me at the end of the fourteen days there was absolutely no hope, I thanked them as sincerely as I knew how for all they had done. I told them, however, that I could not give up on my wife because the Great Physician, the Lord Jesus Christ, was not through with her case.

They told me, "Rev. Williams, if your wife gets well, it will have to be God who does it because she is beyond human help."

Although medical doctors gave me no hope that Pam would live, I am very grateful for the hospitals she was in and for the nursing care she received. We had a blessed opportunity to witness to the doctors and nurses, as well as to people who went to the hospital to visit friends and loved ones. We also witnessed to various patients whom the nurses asked us to visit. Several folks accepted Christ as Saviour, and many others were helped by the Word of God during those days. We trust that the Word is still bearing fruit in their lives.

Many of the preachers who visited their church members in the hospital did not share the Scriptures with them. Some of the people were so terribly ill that we were afraid they might go out into eternity without having heard the Gospel, so we shared some Scriptures with them.

Several expressed surprise over the fact that, while Pam was so near death, we could have the joy of the Lord and be ministering to others. We explained that the Lord Jesus Christ is the One who enables us to have the peace that passes all understanding—even in the midst of severe trial.

After Pam was moved to Acute Care, we were allowed to come and go at any time. We spent many hours a day with her, sitting by her bedside and playing Bible and music tapes. The Gethsemane Quartet, who have been friends of ours for years, graciously gave us some tapes of their songs, and we kept either music or Bible tapes playing in Pam's ear several hours a day.

Up until this time, Pam had not had any therapy. The doctors were so convinced that she was going to die that they would not prescribe therapy. Because of the spasticity of her muscles, her left hand had already begun to turn upward, her feet had turned downward, her neck was stiff, and her arms were tight against her chest in a crossed position.

Since the staff was not administering therapy, I asked them

to at least tell me how to do something to help her. They helped me get her up and tie her in a chair. Then I worked on her body, wiggling her feet and exercising her legs. I rubbed lotion all over her body because her skin had become so dry. We kept Vaseline around her mouth, as the four-pronged instrument that allowed her to breathe caused the sides of her mouth to split and bleed. In fact, Pam still has a scar on her bottom lip from it.

I was glad Pam could not see how she looked; she would have been so embarrassed. To keep her feet from turning down any further, I had purchased some boys' high-top tennis shoes and tied them on her feet. She wouldn't have won any beauty contest, but they surely helped.

After about six weeks, I asked Dr. Shih if we could take Pam back to Denver. I told him that our family physician, Dr. Roland, was willing to fly to Alexandria and discuss Pam's case with him. Since Pam was still in the coma, Dr. Shih said, "Let me think about it, and we'll see how she does."

A day or two later, on a Thursday, he told me, "If your doctor will come here to go over Mrs. Williams' records, you may take her home Monday morning."

I immediately placed a call to one of our dearest friends, Jerry Smith, from Walla Walla, Washington. Jerry and his wife Jane have helped us so much over the years of our ministry.

I knew that Jerry had a Lear Jet, and I felt that he would make it available for us to transport Pam to Denver.

When I called, Jerry was not in. Even his parents did not know how to reach him. They said he was in Hawaii on an extended vacation and didn't want to be bothered.

In the waiting room of the hospital, I dropped to my knees and prayed, "Lord, You know that I need to talk to Jerry. Please help me."

I had hardly gotten off my knees when the phone rang in the waiting room. It was Jerry. "Tom, I was just passing a phone and felt that I ought to call you."

The Spirit of God had reached over to the Hawaiian Islands and touched his heart to call. I almost shouted with joy!

I explained our situation to Jerry, and he said, "Sure, you can use the plane!"

Jerry's pilots flew to Denver, picked up Dr. Roland, and flew to the National Airport in Washington, D.C. After Dr. Roland studied Pam's records with Dr. Shih at the hospital, we rented an ambulance to take Pam to the airport. There Pam and I, along with Phyllis, Penny and Dr. Roland, boarded the plane and left for Denver.

Our son Paul and Bob Criswell (one of the men working with us in our rodeo ministry) drove our motor home across country to Denver, traveling with the Rooneys as they also returned to Denver in their motor home. How we appreciated the Criswells through this trial! Bob, Ethel, Cheryl, Coleen and Clinton have been a tremendous blessing to us. Ethel spent a lot of time helping Pam and trying to encourage her.

When we arrived at the Denver airport, an ambulance from Mercy Hospital met us and took us immediately to the hospital, where Dr. Roland had arranged for Pam to be admitted.

The doctors in Denver began to study Pam's situation. They said that, unless she took a turn for the good within thirty days, there really would not be any hope for her. They ran all the tests that had been run at Alexandria Hospital, including brain scans, an EEG, an arteriogram and others. But they still could not find anything that might explain why she had not come out of the coma. She didn't have any pus pockets, water pockets or any of the things that comatose patients usually have. The doctors were bewildered.

When Pam was still in Alexandria, after I had started praying about taking her back to Denver, she had been on a drug called Dilantin to keep her from having seizures. Before I took her home, though, I wanted to find out if she would still have the seizures if we took her off that medication. Dilantin tends to cause depression and has other side effects, and I felt that Pam would do better without it.

I asked Dr. Shih how long it would take to get the Dilantin out of her system if we were to stop giving it. He said it would take about ninety-six hours to lose its effect. Since Pam was still in the hospital, they could watch her; so I asked Dr. Shih to stop the Dilantin. If she were going to have another seizure, I wanted her to have it in the hospital, as they would know what to do for her.

Pam didn't have any more Dilantin while she was at Alexandria... and the Lord wonderfully kept her from having seizures.

Except for Dr. Roland, all of her doctors in the Denver hospital wanted to put her back on Dilantin; but because of the side effects, I told them I would just trust the Lord not to let her have any more seizures.

At the end of two weeks in Denver, when it seemed that nothing more could be done for Pam, I told Dr. Roland, "I believe I would like to take Pam home and try to take care of her myself."

Although he didn't think I was wise to take on such a monumental task, Dr. Roland agreed to let me try. The nurses taught me how to feed Pam through the tube that was in her nose and how to run the catheter. The therapists in Denver had worked some with Pam, and they allowed me to work along with them so I could learn therapy. One of the therapists, Lel Fickett, was a Christian young lady who agreed to come to our home twice a week to teach me new therapy and make sure I was doing the therapy correctly on Pam. How much we appreciated her help and encouragement!

After staying at the Clarks' home for two weeks, we moved back to our home, a forty-foot Continental Trailways coach which had been converted to a motor home. There we spent the next seventeen months. Many folks wanted me to put my wife in a rehabilitation center, but Pam had always been dependent upon my love and affection for strength and encouragement, and I knew that she needed her home and family more now than ever before. I believed by that time Pam could hear what we were saying, and she seemed to respond to my voice in particular. So I told everyone that I simply must keep Pam at home and take care of her there.

How grateful we are to the doctors, nurses and friends who sacrificed their time and effort to help us through the long vigil of nearly four months from the time she got sick until the doctors believed that perhaps she was out of the coma! They could not tell for sure because there still was no outward response. She could neither speak nor move any of her limbs. Then she began to wiggle a finger, then a toe. One day she blurted out, "NO!" And then she didn't say anything else for days and days. One time she said "strawberry." Then another long period of silence.

It went on like that until August 18. And for the first time in more than five months, Pam spoke in response to a question, and a new life began for us.

I was holding a revival meeting in Knoxville, Tennessee, and our motor home was parked at the Knoxville Baptist Tabernacle, where Dr. Bob Bevington is pastor.

About 9:30 p.m. our son Paul had come to our bedroom to tell us good night. Paul had given his mother a little stuffed dog a few weeks earlier, and he placed it on the bed beside her each night. We had named it Rainbow because of the different colors in the fabric.

As he had done many times, Paul picked up the dog and asked, "Mother, what is this dog's name?"

And as best as she could, Pam answered, "Rainbow."

I'm sure I don't have to tell you there were much rejoicing and tears! She said our names that night for the first time since March 9. The long vigil was over, and she began to talk some on a regular basis. Hope shined in our hearts brighter than ever, hope that someday she really would be well.

CHAPTER 5

It Can Be Done

How many times someone says, "It just can't be done! I can't do it! There isn't any way we could do that!"

I have heard these statements many times, often in referring to the care of loved ones who are ill. But in many cases, it was not a matter of the impossible; it was a matter that someone was not willing to sacrifice what was necessary in order to do what needed to be done.

I had started back preaching in July after Pam became ill in March, and we took her with us in the motor home and cared for her. As a family we vowed to do all we could to see her get well.

I would be the first to admit that it isn't easy to care for an invalid. And although I loved my wife very dearly, there were many times that I exercised her body out of duty, knowing that was her only hope of ever being anywhere close to normal.

It was hard to keep on day after day, hearing Pam scream from pain as I administered therapy to her. It was hard for the children to do their schoolwork with Pam screaming in the next room. But since we traveled all the time, they had to do their schooling by correspondence; so they had no other choice.

I worked with Pam several hours a day on therapy, regardless of where we were. Every joint in her body had to be moved each day, causing her intense pain. Many people didn't understand what was happening. When we were in trailer parks between meetings, the people next to us would hear her crying and wonder what was happening. In motels, we sometimes had to explain to the people in the rooms next to ours what was happening. I'm sure they thought I was beating my wife. But we kept doing what needed to be done.

I tied Pam to a specially made board and stood her upright on it, giving her the sensation of standing. I turned the board around and around to give her the sensation of spinning and motion. I carried her out to the car and tied her in the seat, driving over mountainous curves so she could get a sensation of movement and motion. I also carried her outside so she could sit in the sunlight each day.

We had to keep a chart of her fluids, measuring everything we gave her to eat or drink, as well as her output. We had to check her pulse rate and blood pressure and take her temperature twice a day. While Pam was in bed, we turned her every two hours to reduce the possibility of bed sores. We had to process all of her food through the blender so it could be forced down the tube in her nose.

When I first started thinking of bringing Pam home from the hospital, I didn't know how to do any of these things. But the staff very patiently worked with me. It was no easy task to learn the procedures and do them, but we did it because of our love and concern for her.

I hope that many folks who read this book will be encouraged to do what is right by their family and loved ones; to encourage them with family love and family surroundings; to take care of a mother or daddy, a wife or husband, or a child who has been left invalid because of a disease or accident. The love and compassion of family members has a great healing effect on folks like this. I am confident that such an atmosphere is one of the major factors in Pam's having progressed as much as she has.

Before Pam's illness, she had beautiful hair that hung

almost to her waist. Gradually most of it fell out—partly because of the illness and partly from lying on it all the time. But thank God, it grew back. It is thicker and healthier now than it was before she became sick. We are so grateful to God for His loving-kindness toward her and toward us.

CHAPTER 6

Step by Step

How I thank God that He gave me a large, physically strong body! It was such a blessing during the time Pam was totally helpless.

In the hospital I lifted her from the bed and put her on the table or cot when the nurses needed to move her from one room to another. The day we took her home from the hospital, I carried her to the car.

When we arrived at the Clarks', where we were to stay for two weeks, I carried her up the stairs and put her on the hospital bed. For the next four months, I carried Pam everywhere she went.

Pam's feet were pointed downward from the lack of therapy while she was in the hospital in Virginia. Doctors and therapists told me that Pam would never again be able to walk unless she had surgery on her feet, but I prayed and asked God to help me bring her feet back to where they were supposed to be without her having surgery.

When I pulled on her feet, I had to hold her knees in such a way that I did not injure them from the tremendous pressure I was applying. I put her knee into my shoulder and reached down with both hands, pulling on one foot at a time. I held it in that position for a long period of time each day, making very little progress, but grateful for even slight results.

At night we put a specially made board in her bed and tied her feet to it. The board was designed to keep her feet from going back to the position they were in before therapy. Little by little her feet began to straighten, even though her toes were still turned downward. We continued to work with her feet until they were back to some semblance of where they belonged. Then we stood her upright beside the bed two or three times a day, forcing her weight down on her feet.

We kept rubbing them to get the blood circulating back up her legs, constantly rubbing upward toward the heart. The children rubbed her legs until they were so tired they could rub no longer. Then I rubbed her legs while they held her upright.

For several months Pam's body was so stiff that she could not bend to sit down. But as we continued working with her, the day finally came that she could sit. Then she was able to sit in a wheelchair.

We were in the area of the Rose Hill Baptist Church, and they asked, "Brother Tom, is there anything you need?"

I replied, "Yes, we desperately need a wheelchair."

A lady in the church had one, and she gladly gave it to us, for which we were grateful.

The wheelchair was one of the hardest things I had to accept. I suppose it was because of pride, but I did not want to admit that my wife was really an invalid and needed a wheelchair. For awhile, I was embarrassed for folks to see Pam in a wheelchair, but I soon overcame my embarrassment and became thankful for it. It was such a wonderful help to us.

I shall never forget the day in September, 1978, when we wheeled Pam down the aisle at the South Sheridan Baptist Church. This was the first time she had been able to attend services there since she came out of the coma. Everyone gave her a standing ovation. How it touched our hearts! We thanked God for the love, friendship and concern of the dear friends at our home church.

We used the wheelchair for almost a year, taking Pam many places she otherwise would not have been able to go. We tried to get her out as much as possible. At first she could not stay in the wheelchair very long, because she was not able to hold up her head for long periods of time. We started with just a few minutes and worked up to an hour, then two hours, then for longer periods until finally we were able to take her to the shopping center and to the grocery store.

It was really a step-by-step process to bring her from being totally crippled and bedridden to becoming somewhat functional. The wheelchair went with us on the airplanes, to churches, through shopping centers and every place Pam went.

Since Pam didn't have the mental ability to know where she should or should not go, we didn't think it was wise to teach her how to use the wheelchair by herself. It was simply a means of moving her from place to place.

When it was time to start teaching her how to walk, she had to start at the beginning, just as a small child would do—with crawling.

During the day, when we were in various areas for meetings, I spread a huge silk sheet on the floor of people's homes and in church auditoriums so I could work with her. I placed Pam on the sheet, face down. She hated this very much, as the weight of her body pressed against spastic muscles and caused much pain. She cried and cried. It seemed that everything we did in an effort to help Pam actually caused pain; but we knew that we had to hurt her in order to help her.

Unlike a baby, Pam didn't have a natural inclination to get up on her hands and knees and try to crawl. We had to position her that way. Little by little we pulled one knee forward and then the other until we got across the room; then we turned her around and helped her back. After many weeks Pam began to crawl. She never took one step until she had crawled a lot.

After she seemed fairly stable at crawling, we tried to help her walk. First we taught Pam to get out of the wheelchair by herself, then to stand still until she had gained her balance. Little by little she gained enough confidence to try to stand alone—first by leaning against something and then by holding onto us.

To help her start walking, we moved one leg forward, then the other. One of us held her upright while two of us moved her legs. This took place in the hallway of our motor home.

When we felt she was ready to take some steps by herself, we stood in front of her, just like we would stand before a little child, and said, "Come on now, walk to me." But nothing much happened until Christmas Day in 1978.

We had prayed and prayed, "O God, for our Christmas gift this year, please let Pam walk on Christmas Day."

We were at the home of some dear friends, Mr. and Mrs. Lewis Rooney of Miles City, Montana. (They are the parents of Jim Rooney.) Brother Jerry Smith had flown us there as a special Christmas present.

Up to that point, Pam had not called me to her or asked me to do anything since she had become sick. She was just like a small child, letting us do everything for her; she had no initiative to do anything on her own.

On Christmas Day, in the best way she could, Pam said, "Honey, come help me walk." How we rejoiced!

We stood her up, and for the first time, she began to try to walk on her own initiative. I let her hold onto my arm, and she would motivate herself. That was a great day—the day we had prayed for—the day that she, in her own strength, took a step. From that time she began to walk more and more.

We continued to use the wheelchair until April, 1979, as the most she could walk was the length of our motor home, and only then by holding onto things or people.

During the second week of April we were parked at the home of Pastor and Mrs. Al Cockrell in Kansas City. (They now have a church in Tampa, Florida.) While we were there we began to encourage Pam to walk longer distances. First it was just the length of the driveway, then out one driveway and down the street and up another driveway—not just once in the morning, but also in the afternoon. My, we felt such a sense of accomplishment when she was able to walk a hundred yards! I'm sure that a hundred yards probably seemed like the length of the world to her, but it was thrilling to see her progress and be able to walk.

Pam now walks about a mile each day (weather permitting), climbs the doorsteps of our home by herself, and rides her exercycle about a mile each day.

Truly her learning to walk was a step-by-step process, taking hours and hours of encouragement to keep on trying. When it hurt to walk, when she cried because she had to walk, when she did not want to walk, we kept on encouraging her. The children took her for walks; I took her for walks; friends came and walked with her.

Yes, it required much patience, diligence and hard work; but it was worth every minute we spent helping her. And it will be worth it to you, my friend, to help your loved ones or a friend— step by step—to come back from a trial, whether it be an illness, an automobile wreck or some other incident. It is tremendously rewarding to see them walking again.

CHAPTER 7

A Dark Day in Washington

Nine months after Pam became ill, we were in the state of Washington holding a meeting. Our family had made many adjustments, and things seemingly were going along pretty well. Of course, we had our days of depression and our times of difficulties; but all in all, we were doing quite well in our situation.

A couple of our friends, Don Linkem and Dick Crowe, had taken Pam and me to lunch. We were almost back to the motor home when Pam's body suddenly stiffened and her hands rolled in toward each other. Her mouth drew up to one side, her gaze fixed, and she began to gasp for breath. Then she stopped breathing and began to turn blue.

After my initial shock at seeing her in that condition, I realized she was having another seizure—the first one she had had since she went into the coma at the onset of her illness. Hardly believing what I was seeing, I cried out at the top of my voice, "O God, You must help us! You must help us!"

I was so thankful to God that we were just a few minutes away from a hospital. I did a little bit of fancy driving as we whirled around in the street and headed toward the hospital. Don and Dick lunged forward from the back seat and caught Pam and helped her as much as they could, trying to put something in her mouth so she wouldn't chew or choke on her tongue.

When we reached the hospital, I scooped her into my arms and ran into the hospital. The doctors and nurses started working with her immediately. I stayed in the room with Pam while Don and Dick waited outside.

As Pam began to come out of the seizure, she became violently ill. Finally, after an hour or so, she stopped vomiting.

Shortly after we had arrived at the hospital, Dick and Don had called Ron Ulmen, pastor of the church where we were holding meetings, and told him about Pam. Pastor Ulmen called the hospital later to see how she was doing. We surely appreciated the concern of Pastor Ulmen and his people—not only that day, but all the other times they expressed kindness to us and prayed so earnestly for us in the new trial that we were facing.

The doctors kept Pam at the hospital for a couple of hours to make sure she was not going to have another seizure; then they put her on Dilantin and sent us home.

Needless to say, my heart was burdened and sad. She had been doing so well. We had been administering therapy on Pam, the children were getting adjusted in school, and we had started back traveling. Not knowing how much Pam's seizure would set us back in the progress we all had made—or if she would be more subject to having seizures—I called Dr. Roland in Denver. He said, "Tom, we just don't know. She could have one a day, one a week, one a month, or she could have several in one day. We'll just have to wait and see what's going to transpire now."

We began to pray earnestly that the Lord in His mercy and according to His will would lift this burden from us and would not add to the load we already carried.

I was scheduled to go to Hawaii and preach and also have a time of relaxation and vacation in just about a week, but I didn't know whether Pam should be flying. I didn't know but what the altitude, pressure in the airplane, travel or the long trip might trigger another seizure. We decided to go and just trust the Lord.

During our two weeks in Hawaii, we took great care to keep her away from the lanai (porch) or other places where she might get hurt in case she had another seizure.

Pam was taking two Dilantin capsules each day, but that did not necessarily mean she would not have another seizure. The doctor had told us that, if she had another one, we should lay her on her back, tilt her head backward just a little, put one hand underneath her jawbone and pull up on it to give her breathing passage as much clearance as possible.

Every time she jerked or moved in her sleep, I jumped straight up in bed to see if she was all right. Sitting in an airplane or in a car, I constantly watched her out of the corner of my eye to make sure she was doing okay.

Even with our constant vigil over Pam, she had another seizure about a month later. We noticed that there seemed to be some connection between the seizures and Pam's time of month, so we started making sure she got plenty of rest during that time, hoping to ward off future seizures. But they continued to recur. We praise God that all but one happened in private. Some were in the car; others, in our motor home. The one in public was in Kansas City. Pam was with a very close friend of hers, Janie Cockrell. Janie had taken Pam to an exercise class. Of course, Pam really could not do the exercises properly, but we thought it might be good therapy for her to go and at least try.

As they were going through some of the exercises, Pam started having a seizure. The instructor of the class was familiar with seizures, so she knew what to do.

We had prayed and prayed that God would take away the seizures and that Pam wouldn't be afflicted with them. She was still taking the Dilantin, but it was not controlling the seizures. We didn't know what to do.

We had gone to the Rooneys' ranch again so I could help

round up the cattle. This was something I really enjoyed doing, and it gave me a tremendous change of pace. Before I went there, I mentioned to someone that the Rooneys live sixty-five miles from any town. Surprised that I was taking Pam to a place that far away, she replied, "There is a community store, isn't there?"

"No."

"No place to buy gas?"

"No. The ranch is sixty-five miles from Miles City, Montana, where they do all their shopping and trading. There's not a store, gas station or anything between the ranch and the city except other ranches."

So there we were, sixty-five miles from town, from a hospital, from a doctor; and it was time for Pam to have another seizure. The Lord spoke to my heart and said, "Tom, you have been asking Me to take away the seizures; now where is your faith? I want you to take Pam off the medicine."

My first inclination was to question God as I wondered why He had waited until we were totally out of reach of the hospital before He told me to stop the medicine. Why couldn't He have told me that while we were parked at a big city church where there are hospitals all around? But He didn't choose to do that.

I said, "Okay, Father, if that's the way it has to be, then I'll do it."

I told Penny, my youngest daughter, "Honey, we're going to stop giving your mother the Dilantin. We're going to trust the Lord."

Hardly believing what she was hearing, she startlingly replied, "But, Daddy, it's time for Mother to have another seizure."

"I know, but God has asked me to take away the medicine. I must do as He says."

God blessed our obedience in spite of our wavering faith. Even as I write this book, I can't help but cry and rejoice in thanksgiving to God for taking away the seizures. That was in May, 1979.

Month after month we rejoiced over the fact that she was not having seizures. In fact, Pam did not have another seizure for more than a year. We were surprised and disappointed when the seizures returned; but at the same time, we were grateful to God that she had gone so long without having one.

My heart goes out to folks who have seizures. God taught me so many lessons during those times. How much more I pray for those who are sick! How much more I am able to sympathize and identify with those who have some kind of physical ailment! Until our experience with Pam's seizures, I don't suppose I ever really thought much about the many folks who have them, but I certainly do now. I pray for them on a regular basis and ask God to control and to free them from the seizures.

Yes, it was a dark day in Washington the day Pam had her seizure in January, 1979, but God led us out of the darkness and into the light as He delivered Pam from the seizures for such a long period of time. Oh, what a wonderful God we have! How merciful He is! I truly praise Him for answering prayer for His children.

Pam has not yet been totally healed; her mind has not yet fully returned to where she can do things that she used to do; and she is not mentally capable of being the wife and mother that I know she would long to be, if she were well. I am sure that many of you who read this book will still be going through trials. Let me share with you a couple of verses that have been a tremendous encouragement to me as we continue in our trial.

Proverbs 23:17,18 says, "Let not thine heart envy sinners: but be thou in the fear of the Lord all the day long. For surely there is an end; and thine expectation shall not be cut off."

Thank God that there is an end—regardless of the trial. If God does not end it in this physical realm, He will end

it when He receives us in Glory, where we shall be made
whole and have a body like unto His glorious body. Yes, there
is an end. Thank God, there will be an end to the seizures.
Thank God, there will be an end to the affliction of Pam's
physical malady—if not in this life, then in that blessed life
to come.

And there will be an end to your trial, dear friend, regardless of how severe it may be. Remember the verse: "For surely there is an end; and thine expectation shall not be cut off."

CHAPTER 8

Pam's Progress

From the day Pam left the hospital, during the time we lived in the Clarks' home, and even after we moved back into our motor home, she made some progress. At first, the progress was tremendously slow. For days and weeks we watched for every sign of improvement.

Finally, Pam wiggled a toe, then a finger, then batted an eye. That was progress. We would tell her, "You are making progress. Oh, you are doing great!" We were hoping she was hearing and understanding us.

Encouragement is such a blessing to anybody, and especially to folks who are sick or in a coma. It is some of the best medicine they can possibly receive.

We encouraged Pam in every way we could. We bragged on her every day. Even if the progress was something very simple, we would tell her how well she was doing, how she was going to make it, how God was helping her and that folks were praying for her. Every time someone called and asked about her, I told Pam about the call. I read every letter to her, hoping she could understand how much people were concerned.

Just Like a Baby

Pam had to go through every step that a child goes through.

Moms, remember how excited you were when your baby did things for the first time? How you could hardly wait for your husband to get home so you could tell him what the baby had done that day?

Dads, remember how excited you were when your wife came home from town and you told her something the baby had done for the first time?

That's the way it is when someone in Pam's situation starts doing things again for the first time after a coma or long illness. We experienced the same initial thrill when we saw her making progress.

When a baby begins to crawl and pull up, we have to put away things that we didn't have to put away before. When a baby starts walking, we have to protect him from climbing or falling down the stairs; we have to be careful to close doors or gates to keep him *out of* certain places and *in* certain rooms or areas. We constantly had to watch Pam and protect her in all these areas once she came out of the coma and started relearning various things.

Diapers by the Dozen

Like a baby, Pam went through the diaper stage. We had a catheter on her, but because of infections and other problems, it became necessary to remove it. Since she did not have control over those bodily functions, we began to diaper her. We bought diapers by the case—twenty-four dozen at a time.

It took fourteen months to potty-train Pam. We would work with her just like a parent would work with a baby, putting her on the potty and encouraging her to use the bathroom. We praised her when she did, and we tried to be patient with her when she didn't. Many times we would leave her there for half an hour or so, and she would fuss the entire time. When we finally let her get up, she would soil the diaper almost immediately. You probably know what a chore it is to constantly change a baby's diaper. Just imagine how much more difficult it was to change an adult!

I'm sure Pam does not remember those discouraging times, but that's the way it was for fourteen long months before she would tell us. Then, just like a child tells when he needs to use the bathroom, Pam finally started to tell us. There were times when she would forget, but we were so grateful for the progress she was making.

Then came the day that she finally learned to use the restroom every time. What a tremendous help that was!

When I took Pam to the airport, shopping center or other places by myself, we faced some very interesting moments. We would be in the airport or in a shopping center, and Pam would say, "Honey, I have to go to the bathroom."

I was in quite a predicament. She was in a wheelchair and could not walk well enough to go to the ladies' room alone; and of course I could not take her to the men's room.

I remember one time in the Atlanta airport when Pam told me that she needed to use the restroom. I talked to a stewardess, but she didn't want to take Pam. She was afraid that she might hurt her and that I might sue the airlines.

One of the airline officials finally agreed to take her; but when she got Pam to the bathroom, she changed her mind. She, too, was afraid she might hurt Pam and that I might sue the airlines. I tried to assure both of them that I wouldn't sue, but they still wouldn't take her.

By this time Pam was getting desperate. Finally the lady noticed a 747 jet at one of the gates. "No one is on that plane right now; it's not ready to leave yet. You can take your wife to the restroom there."

So she let us go down the walkway and into the airplane so Pam could use the restroom.

It seemed that we especially had problems when Pam had to use the restroom on airplanes—not only that time, but practically every time we flew.

If you could have seen Pam and me both squeezed into one

of those restrooms, you would have chuckled. They are so *tiny*. The stewardesses could hardly believe it when I would open the door and Pam and I both would come out of the same restroom.

Once when Phyllis took Pam to the restroom, one lady said, "Did you see two ladies come out of the airplane restroom? I don't believe it. They both came out of the same one!"

Yes, we have had some very interesting times—as well as some very embarrassing times. Pam sometimes would forget to tell us—even when she was in public or while sitting in the church pew. Of course, that always created a problem. But we just thanked God that she was progressing as well as she was. What a blessing when Pam had progressed to the point that she could go to the bathroom by herself!

Learning to Eat

Pam's coordination wasn't very good because the motor control in her brain had been damaged as a result of the illness. I clearly remember when we started trying to teach her how to eat after she came out of the coma.

The first time we put a spoon in her hand, she did exactly what babies do—she dumped the food halfway between the plate and her mouth. She would put food in her ear, in her hair, on the table or floor—everywhere except in her mouth. She would fork at things and miss them. Then she would try to get the food with a spoon, but she didn't know how to use something to push the food onto the spoon; so she would shove it off the edge of the plate.

A parent expects these types of problems in rearing children, but we also had to accept them as a way of life for Pam during that learning period. And, like everything else, we had to learn patience so we could properly respond to her.

Brushing Her Teeth

Pam didn't have any idea how to use a toothbrush or even

which toothbrush was hers. Sometimes she tried to brush her teeth without any toothpaste; at other times she used two or three times as much as she needed. We had to make sure she used toothpaste, that she put the lid back on the tube, that she brushed the front *and* the back teeth, that she rinsed her toothbrush, and that she put it back where it belonged when she was finished.

Discipline

Pam also went through the spitting stage. When I insisted that she do certain things she didn't want to do or eat things she didn't like, she would spit on me or on something close by. And, just like a child, she had to be disciplined. I didn't spank her very hard, but I did have to discipline her for wrongdoing. It was very difficult for me to spank my wife; but, of course, I had to remind myself that, apart from discipline, she would do things that might be harmful to herself as well as to others.

I had to treat her like a child part of the time and like an adult at other times. This was very hard on her, on the children and on me; but if she were going to continue to progress, then these things had to be done.

Dressing Herself

Remember the times your youngsters came out of the bedroom half-dressed, clothes buttoned crooked, put on backward—or sometimes with no clothes on at all? Well, Pam did the same thing. Sometimes she would have her dress buttoned, but it would be buttoned wrong; at other times she would put her clothes on backward and wonder why she couldn't find the buttons.

With much effort, Pam finally learned to put on her shoes again. It took many months to teach her to tie her shoestrings. It would have been much easier to always let her wear slip-ons, but the others seemed to give better support.

Little by little, she is improving, but she still cannot fully dress herself. We just continue working with her. One of her most recent accomplishments has been to put in her earrings. This was hard to learn because of her limited coordination.

Learning to Tell Time

It took weeks to teach Pam how to put her watch around her wrist and fasten it. And it took much longer to teach her how to tell time.

Because of brain damage, Pam did not have any sense of responsibility, and she constantly misplaced her watch. Just like a child, she left it wherever she took it off—in the bed, in the bathtub, on the floor, in the living room or kitchen, or anywhere else.

We had the same problem trying to keep up with her glasses. Before Pam's illness she had worn contact lenses; but since she could not take care of the lenses in her condition, she had to start back wearing glasses. She would get annoyed with them and take them off. We were as likely to find them in the kitchen or in the living room as on her face. Sometimes we found them on the floor or in her wheelchair. We very patiently worked with her and tried to emphasize to her the importance of wearing them so she could see better.

Her lack of responsibility toward her watch and her glasses reminded me of our son Tim's lack of responsibility when he was young. When Tim was two years old, we discovered that something was wrong with his eyes, and he had to wear glasses. As you can imagine with a child that age, we found his glasses in the sandbox, in the toy box, in the backyard, everywhere. We never knew where he would leave them.

New Inventions

All during the early stages of Pam's recovery, we had to invent things that would help her make progress. On the hand where her fingers were stiff and straight, we used a device that the therapist had made to help her close her hand. It fastened around her wrist and had leather finger-tips with rubber bands attached to them. We used another device at night to curve her fingers and hold them in place. On the hand where her fingers were curled under, we used a device to hold open her fingers.

We didn't depend on the ingenuity of others alone; we tried to think of everything we possibly could to help her.

We bought a toy gun with a strong trigger and taught her to squeeze it. This not only exercised and strengthened her hand and arm muscles, but it was a source of entertainment as our children played with her.

To improve Pam's coordination we tied a rubber band on a rubber ball and attached it over her bed, teaching her to hit the ball and try to catch it while it was still moving.

We tried to teach her how to write, but her coordination has not been good enough to write properly. I talked to a therapist, and she suggested that we concentrate on help-ing her learn things, such as reading, that would make life more enjoyable for her, yet not frustrate her with trying to write.

Following her advice, we set out to teach her other things. Pam learned to spell quite well, to say her "A,B,C's" and to count to one hundred by fives, tens and by ones. She can read road signs, simple books and *some* letters that people send her. She can solve a few simple math problems.

It thrills her, and us, that she is able once again to think of things on her own, to say and do things on her own. It is so wonderful. When she does something for herself, it's twice as rewarding than our doing it for her. And it en-courages her to try even harder.

Folks have asked me, "Tom, will Pam ever again be like she was before the illness?"

I don't know the answer to that question, but we just

continue to work with her and to commit our situation to the Lord.

Others have asked, "Are you still glad you went to Israel, even though Pam got sick over there?"

Yes, I am. She could have contracted meningitis anywhere.

Pam and I had such a wonderful time those last few days before her illness. I would not trade those precious moments for anything.

Our hearts were so blessed, and I can understand my Bible so much better. Truly, I am glad that we decided to go. It was the thrill of a lifetime!

Many have asked, "Brother Williams, don't you get weary?"

Yes, I do get weary. And it is difficult at times to keep going. But, oh, the reward of seeing her happy, encouraged and doing things on her own again!

Pam's progress has been painstakingly slow, but she has made progress. Sometimes it's easy to become discouraged with Pam and think she will never be well. Then we remember her condition when she first came out of the coma and realize just how far she has come. This gives us new strength, new vision and new determination to get back in the battle and try to teach her something else. I just praise the Lord that He has brought us this far.

If you have a problem child or if you have a mother, daddy or friend that is in a situation similar to Pam's, just remember: progress may seem painstakingly slow; but if there's any sign of improvement at all, they are making progress. Just continue to love and encourage them.

Let me ask you, as I close this chapter, to consider how long it has been since you thanked God that you could:

1. Get out of bed.
2. Walk correctly, or walk at all.
3. Look in the mirror and recognize yourself.
4. Feed yourself.
5. Dress yourself.

6. Tie your shoes.

7. Hear and understand.

8. Bathe yourself.

9. Leave home and remember how to get back.

10. Help someone else.

Have you told your wife, your husband, your children, your parents, that you love them and appreciate them? Just love them for what they are and not for what you think they ought to be or wish they were!

CHAPTER 9

Things That Have Happened

God has used the story of Pam's illness and miraculous events to touch the hearts and lives of many people.

A Child's Faith

Let me tell you about a little six-year-old boy named David Guy. Although David was just a young boy, God had answered many of his prayers.

At the time Pam became ill, David lived in Alexandria, Virginia. His dad, Alden Guy, was a colonel at the Pentagon. They were (and still are) members of the Fairfax Baptist Temple, where Bud Calvert is pastor; so David heard the Word of God from the time he was very young.

David had a tender heart toward the Lord; and by the time he was six years old, he already felt that God had called him to preach. He wanted to walk forward in church and let the pastor and the church folks know about his decision, but his dad thought he was too young. Finally, after David persisted in telling his dad that God had called him to preach, he was allowed to go forward. When he did, he not only told Brother Calvert that God had called him to preach, but he also told the pastor he was glad that God had answered his prayer and spoken to his dad's heart to let him make public his decision. His simple, childlike faith brought results.

Through the various announcements and prayer meetings at Fairfax Baptist Temple, David learned that Pam was very sick. About six o'clock the morning after David went forward, he went into the bathroom where Colonel Guy was shaving. David looked up at him and asked, "Daddy, are you going to the hospital today to see Brother Tom?"

Surprised to see David, he replied, "Yes, I am, son. You are up mighty early this morning."

"Dad, I have been up praying."

It was six o'clock in the morning, and this little fellow, six years old, had already been up praying!

"Dad, would you tell Brother Tom something for me? Tell him that early this morning when I was praying, the Lord told me to tell Brother Tom that Mrs. Williams is going to be all right."

When Colonel Guy gave me David's message, faith and hope gripped my heart like a vise and gave me something to cling to for many days. I knew about David and some of the prayers God had answered for him; and I truly believed God had impressed on his heart that my wife would get better.

I can remember telling the Lord many nights, "Lord, You can't disappoint a six-year-old boy. You told little David that my wife would be all right. She *must* be all right, Lord."

Even though David was just a little boy, his life and prayers have been a tremendous blessing to me. I just want to take this opportunity to say thank you, David, for praying for my wife and for believing God that Mrs. Williams would be all right. God bless you, David Guy.

The Letter God Used

Just a few weeks before Pam and I traveled to Israel, we went to Hawaii for a few days. Like most tourists, Pam bought postcards and sent them to various family members and friends.

About three weeks after Pam became ill, George and Beth Buckley went to the hospital to visit Pam. Beth handed me a letter, telling me that Pam had sent it to her from Hawaii. I didn't even know Pam had written to her.

From Pam's letter, it was as though she knew that something was going to happen to her. The verses she included in the letter fit the situation just as if someone had searched them out in advance and applied them in her life. Quoting from Psalm 118:16-18, Pam had written:

"The right hand of the Lord is exalted: the right hand of the Lord doeth valiantly. I shall not die, but live, and declare the works of the Lord. The Lord hath chastened me sore: but he hath not given me over unto death."

I don't know if God had impressed these verses on Pam's heart to prepare her for what was about to happen or if He was using them to comfort and encourage her during some trials we were experiencing at that time in the ministry. But I clung to those verses like I clung to little David Guy's prayer. I accepted them as God's assurance to me that Pam would not die.

Dr. Ralph Roland, our Christian doctor in Denver, reminded me of these verses many times. He would walk over to Pam's bed and say, "God's going to let you live, Pam; you're not going to die."

Dr. Roland and I thanked God for those verses again and again.

Pam's Long-awaited Answer to Prayer

Don Warner was an excellent wood worker, a structural engineer, a terrific husband and a good daddy. He was a self-sufficient man in many ways, but he had no time for the Lord Jesus Christ. For many years Don had rejected the Lord and seemingly was unconcerned that he was not a Christian.

Don's wife Judy attended South Sheridan Baptist Church, and the folks there had prayed with her concerning his salvation. Many of us had witnessed to Don, but he would not be saved.

Because of Pam's love and appreciation for Judy and the burden that God had put on her heart, Pam prayed for Don Warner's salvation every day for at least four years. I also prayed for him, but not nearly as faithfully as Pam did.

One day I had an opportunity to tell Don how Pam had prayed for him before she became ill, that regardless of how tired she was, where we were or what she was doing, Pam always prayed for Don Warner before she drifted off to sleep. She would say, "Lord, save Don. Help Judy, and strengthen her."

God heard these prayers, and He used them in a wonderful way to bring Don Warner to Himself.

My pastor, Dr. Ed Nelson, had asked me to preach for the morning worship service the Sunday after we transferred Pam from the Alexandria hospital to the hospital in Denver. As I sat by Pam's bedside at the hospital, God laid on my heart a message entitled "Who's Next?"

Judy had told Don that I would be preaching and thought he might like to hear me. He wouldn't come to the service, but he listened to the message on radio as the morning service was broadcast. That evening he came to church with Judy and the children. Don didn't come forward in the service, but he was wonderfully saved by the grace of God that night.

Don later went to the hospital to see Pam, who was still in a coma. Knowing that she had diligently prayed for his salvation, tears welled up in Don's eyes as he took Pam's hand and said, "You may not hear me or understand me, but I want you to know that I am saved as a result of your being sick."

We were thrilled to see him saved and on his way to Heaven as a result of Pam's illness and our family's trial. To God be the glory, great things He hath done!

From Adultery to Salvation

One night after Pam had awakened from the coma, we were in New York for a revival. Pam was on the platform with me as I shared the testimony of our trial, and God used the story in a wonderful way.

After our testimony that evening, I preached. As I gave the invitation, a lady from the back of the auditorium came down the aisle, weeping profusely. As she came forward, she told the counselor, "I'm living with a man who is not my husband. Look at this dear woman and her husband, what they have been through and are going through, how faithful they have been to each other! And look at me! In perfect health and not even saved!"

She was wonderfully saved that evening and went back and told the man that she was with, "We either get married, or we call it quits. I'm not going to live like this anymore after hearing this story tonight."

Thank God for this tremendous victory—for her repentance from sin and for the home that was established!

Faith to Pray for a Miracle

We told the story of our testimony, and I preached in Dallas, Texas, in Dr. Gary Coleman's church, where we had been a number of times. The people's response was tremendous. Many decisions were made for the Lord, lives were changed, and hearts were touched. There was hardly a dry eye in the whole auditorium.

A few days after the meeting, we received a six-page letter from one of the couples who had heard us tell the story. They told me that their baby had become violently ill and had to be taken to the hospital. After the doctors examined the child, they broke the devastating news to the parents that their precious baby had bacterial meningitis and would be dead by morning.

The couple looked at each other and said, "This is the same

disease Pam had. If God answered prayer for Tom Williams, then He will answer prayer for us."

They knelt in the waiting room of the hospital and began to pray like we had done. They prayed all night, crying out to the Lord on behalf of their little one. The next morning the doctor told them, "I don't understand, but the crisis has passed. You can take the baby home."

What a wonderful letter of praise and thanksgiving to God for His mercy and kindness in answering their prayer! They closed the letter by saying: "Brother Tom, thank you for taking Pam around the country and sharing her testimony. We would not have had the faith to pray and believe God if you hadn't recently been here and given your testimony of how God had answered your prayers concerning Pam. Thank you, Brother Tom, for being willing to be used of the Lord."

Strength to Continue

In Parsippany, New Jersey, I held a number of meetings for my friend, Pastor Jack Keep. The folks at Parsippany Baptist Church have been so kind to us. We thank God for them. Many of the folks there have bought cassette tapes of my messages. One lady shared our testimony tape with her neighbor, whose three-year-old son had incurable cancer. The little boy was in intense pain, and doctors offered the parents no hope that their child would live. The mother was near exhaustion from having taken care of him for so long, and she was about to break under the physical and emotional strain of watching him slowly die.

After she received our tape, she began to play it every morning. She wrote to us from time to time to keep us informed about how God had used our situation in their lives. In one of the letters she told me:

> Brother Williams, thank you so much for making the tape of your family's testimony. How I thank God for it! He knew just what I needed. I play your tape every

morning, and it gets me through every day of our trial. Also, my husband has started going to church. I just wanted to let you know that God has used your testimony in our lives to meet some tremendous needs.

Airborne and Heavenbound

Pam, the children and I went to Hawaii in January, 1979, to try to get some much needed rest and to see if Pam could remember anything at all about some of the things we had seen and places we had visited on our previous trip to Hawaii. We thank God that she seemed to remember a few of them.

On our way home aboard Continental Airlines, one of the stewardesses stopped to speak to me. "I noticed that something is wrong with your wife, and I was wondering what the problem is."

Since she wasn't really busy at the time, I asked her to sit down. I related to her the story of Pam's illness, our trial, and how the Lord had blessed in a tremendous way in answering prayer and bringing Pam as far back as He had. We were rejoicing in the Lord in being able to share this testimony.

Another stewardess had stopped by and was listening. Soon one of the stewardesses asked, "Do you ever put out tapes?"

"Yes, we have several. Some of them are distributed through our monthly tape ministry, and many others are sold at our meetings."

"I think I've heard one of your tapes. What is your name?"

When I told her, she said, "I was saved through one of your tapes. A man in our airlines has passed your tapes all the way through Continental Airlines up here in the Northwest." (I found out that the man was Brother Meador from Pastor Ron Ulmen's church in Puyallup, Washington.)

Several of the stewardesses came up to us and said they had heard the tape. They were so thrilled to see Pam and me in person and were amazed that we had continued to love and serve the Lord through such an ordeal. Some of them told me they were going to go to church and hear the Gospel and were going to get some more tapes and listen to them. I trust that many more of them have been saved.

A Marriage Restored

While we were in Kansas City, Missouri, holding a meeting for Pastor Al Cockrell at the Tri-City Baptist Church, Mr. Dick Bott, owner of a Christian radio station there, asked us to come and share our testimony on his talk show. For about an hour or so I told what God had done and was doing in our lives and the trial that we were experiencing.

We received a number of calls that morning, and many people said, "I'll never complain again about my petty discomforts and the little things in life that have agitated me."

One lady called and said she would never again be guilty of bickering with her husband but would rejoice in the health and the goodness that God had given them.

About three or four days after the talk show, a man and woman attended a meeting at another church where I was preaching. They came to me after the service, and the woman said, "You don't know us, but we were listening to the radio the other day when you were telling about Pam's illness. My husband and I were separated at the time because we just couldn't get along.

"I was not aware that my husband was listening to the broadcast, and he didn't know that I was. Immediately after the talk show, I went to the apartment where my husband was staying. He wasn't there...but I found out later that he had left to come looking for me. Since that time, we have found one another...and have really found ourselves."

She told her husband, "I want us to get back together. I will love you for what you are and not for what I think you ought to be."

He expressed to her the same sentiment, and they got back together.

During that week, they came to the meetings several times. Before I left the city, they told me, "We now have a home and a marriage because of the trial of your life, the testimony of your love for your wife and the way you have taken care of her and have given yourself for her."

Back to the Lord

Pam is the oldest of three girls in her family; Peggy is next to Pam; and Annette is the youngest. Peggy had been saved through our ministry while we were living in California, but she had gotten away from the Lord and was not living for Him. In fact, at that time she really didn't seem to have any desire to serve Him.

When Peggy heard that Pam was so ill and was near the point of death, she turned back to the Lord and started once again going to church, reading her Bible and praying.

She has written to us many times, telling us that she is praying for us, and she has expressed constant interest in Pam. It thrills our hearts to know that God has used our testimony in the life of someone who is so near and dear to us. We can only say, Praise His holy name!

God's Sufficient Grace

One of the ladies of our church in Denver came to me one day and said, "Brother Williams, I had always wondered if it were possible for a man to fulfill God's words in Ephesians 5 and love his wife as his own body. Pam has been sick almost two years now, and I've noticed how you have cared for her. Brother Williams, I now believe that it's possible, for I have seen one man who loves his wife as his own body."

I don't tell this story to brag on Tom Williams, but to brag on God, whose grace is sufficient for every trial and in every situation.

I thank God for the many people who have heard my marriage seminar and have written, saying, "I now believe with all my heart that you love Pam like you say in your marriage seminars that you love her."

Multitudes of Others

Other letters have come from all over the world, saying, "Brother Williams, what a tremendous blessing your life and testimony have been to us! What an encouragement it has been to see the power and the grace of God in your life—to see living proof of what we know to be true and what you have been preaching for years!"

Countless times on airplanes folks have asked me what was wrong with Pam. We have shared the testimony of God's love and mercy with passengers, stewardesses, pilots and people in the airport. We have been in church after church where there was not a dry eye in the entire auditorium as we told about the many hours, the many days, the long months of our trial. Literally thousands of people have told us, "Thank you. We have heard many great sermons, but we have never seen a sermon like we have seen today of the answer to prayer, of the strength and the grace of God."

We could tell of the lady in California whose husband had not spoken for years. He is mentally alert and can understand everything people say, but he can't speak a word. He can't walk, and he has very little use of his hands. This man's wife was comforted as I spoke to her, for she felt that I really understood her situation.

We could tell about many of the multiplied thousands that God has strengthened, helped and blessed for His glory through Pam's illness.

Miracle of the Seventh Floor

I have taken Pam back to both hospitals—the one in Denver, Colorado, and the one in Alexandria, Virginia—to show the doctors and nurses what God has done in her life. At both hospitals the Lord was glorified as the nurses and doctors said, "God has worked a miracle!"

They were completely amazed at Pam's recovery. One nurse screamed out loud when she saw Pam; it was as though she had seen a ghost. "I never expected to see you walking around and looking like this!"

Mrs. Riffel, one of the nurses in charge of taking care of Pam at the Mercy Hospital in Denver, told me, "Mr. Williams, Pam is the miracle of the seventh floor."

Many nurses have said that Pam was the only person they knew who had been as sick as she had been—and had lived.

Judy Graham was a therapist who came with Lel Fickett to our home on several occasions. Lel and our family would pray and witness to Judy about her salvation and tell her that she needed to receive Jesus Christ as her Saviour, but she would always put it off. Several months later, when our family had supper with Judy and two other therapists, she looked across the table and said, "Mr. Williams, I have been saved since I last saw you."

She went on to say that the main factor that brought her to Christ was our family's love for Mrs. Williams: "I knew it had to be a God-given love."

Once again, we just want to say, Thank You, Lord, for using our lives, our family for Your glory to meet the needs of people around the country through our trial.

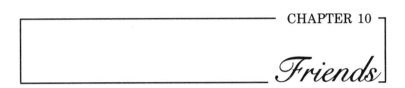

CHAPTER 10

A true friend is a wonderful blessing from God, and He has blessed us many times through the thousands of friends He has given us.

Because of my work in evangelism, Pam and I were apart much of the time before her illness. But God blessed our willingness to sacrifice for Him, and countless numbers of friends stood by us in our hour of need.

From Japan, Brazil, the Philippine Islands, Australia, Germany—from all over the world, missionaries sent telegrams to us at the hospital, saying they were praying for Pam. So many people called the hospital that a special operator was appointed just to take our calls.

Pastors wrote and sent packets of letters from their people who had taken time to write a note to us. We spent hours reading those precious letters. Tears streamed down our faces as we realized that so many people remembered and cared during those hours of the long wait.

I cannot possibly list here all those who wrote, called and cared; but I would like to mention just a few.

I am so grateful for Pastor and Mrs. Pat Upshaw and members of the Rose Hill Baptist Church in Alexandria, Virginia, who provided food for our family every other day and allowed us to leave the motor home parked at the church for weeks. Pastor Upshaw spent much time with me at the hospital and took my place in the waiting room so I could leave and get some rest. I felt better knowing that someone was there, waiting for any message that might come from the Intensive Care Unit.

We were allowed to see Pam for a half hour every three or four hours, but the staff kindly permitted us to see her a little more frequently, since they didn't think she would live very long.

It would take pages to record the kindness, concern and love shown by Pastor and Mrs. Bud Calvert and the members of Fairfax Baptist Temple in Fairfax, Virginia. They alternated days with Rose Hill Baptist and made sure our family had plenty to eat.

Brother Calvert also stood by us during the long hours of waiting to find out what was wrong with Pam, to see if she would get well or if she would drift out into eternity. He and Pastor Upshaw prayed, wept and stood by us for many weeks.

Brother Calvert's church called a special prayer meeting that first night while we kept vigil by Pam's bed to see if she would make it through the first twenty-four hours. It was Bud Calvert and his people who gave money to pay the first part of Pam's hospital bill.

The lady in the business office had sent word that she needed to see me. When I reached her office, she said, "Mr. Williams, you don't have medical insurance, do you?"

"No, ma'am, I don't."

"This bill is going to run $16,000 minimum if she lives very long at all. Right now it's running $1,600 a day. You must come up with some money, at least $3,000, by three o'clock this afternoon."

I assured her that I would speak to my Father about the situation.

My Heavenly Father had promised to supply our needs, and I was sure that He would.

When I returned upstairs, Brother Calvert was there. He asked, "Where have you been, Tom?"

"Down at the business office."

"What did they want?"

"Money. To be exact, $3,000 by three o'clock this afternoon."

Brother Calvert grinned. "My church would like to take care of that amount for you." And he gave me a check for $3,500—the $3,000 we needed, plus an additional $500. Isn't that just like the Lord!

Even as I write this book, tears of gratitude stream down my face as I think of the kindness of Brother Calvert and his people.

Pastor Calvert's church became the receiving station for the money that came in from all over the world to help with the huge expense. They kept a record of the money received and sent a receipt to the person or church sending the money. They also wrote checks to the hospital and kept abreast of the bill day by day.

Let me pause here to say that some of you probably feel I was negligent in not having medical insurance. I don't think there's anything wrong with having insurance. In fact, I believe most people should have it. But *my* reason for not having any is that God had very clearly spoken separately to my heart and to Pam's in 1962 and told us we were not to have medical insurance. Ever since, God had miraculously paid all our medical bills, and I had no reason to doubt that He would do the same again—even though this bill would far exceed any we had ever incurred. Our Heavenly Father again proved His faithfulness and met our needs.

Another person I would like to mention is the man who was our pastor, Dr. Ed Nelson, along with his wife and fellow members of the South Sheridan Baptist Church in Denver. Soon after hearing that Pam was sick, Dr. Nelson flew in from Denver. Then Pastor Nelson, Pastor Calvert and I entered Pam's room, anointed her with oil and prayed over her.

We believe that, when the Spirit of God leads, we can follow the teaching of James 5 and expect God to do something. In Pam's case and in many others, we have seen miraculous results by simply praying and claiming the promise God gave. Dr. Nelson stayed a few hours, then returned home to his busy schedule.

In a couple of days he called and asked, "Tom, how are things going?"

I told him what little I knew about Pam's condition.

He asked, "How are finances?"

I replied, "I just returned from the business office. I need to come up with another $4,000 because the $3,500 has already been used."

"Tom, that won't be any problem. We took an offering for you last night, and it was $4,120."

What a blessing and thrill to my heart! How we thank God for our pastor and for all our friends at our home church! Then and in the following months, they met a tremendous need in our lives.

Another friend I would like to acknowledge is Dr. Ralph Roland, our family doctor. Dr. Roland advised me by telephone while Pam was still in Alexandria. Then when it seemed that she was not making any further progress, I called and asked if he would come to the Alexandria hospital, look at Pam's medical records, talk to her doctors and then fly back to Denver with Pam and me.

When Pam was moved to the hospital in Denver, Dr. Roland diligently cared for her and was available to us by telephone day and night.

After I took Pam home and began taking care of her (with the help of others, including many from South Sheridan Baptist Church), Dr. Roland came almost every day to see how Pam was doing and to check the records we were keeping of her fluid intake and output, her temperature, heart rate and other things. Without Dr. Roland's help, it would have been impossible to keep Pam at home. How I thank God for him and for his wife Carol, who so unselfishly shares him with others!

I also thank Carl and Christy Clark, some of our closest personal friends, who opened their home to us, put a hospital bed in one room and allowed us to stay there for the first two weeks Pam was out of the hospital.

Carl worked diligently to get the hospital bed in the house. He put ladders up the back of his house, tied ropes to each end of the bed, and had others help him pull it onto the balcony. Then they took it through the sliding doors of their bedroom and worked it down the hall and into the room that we used.

Their diligence in getting the bed into the house reminded me of the four men in Bible days who brought their sick friend to Jesus so he could be healed (Mark 2:2-5).

God gave Carl and Christy special grace during those days as a constant flow of people poured in and out of their house—nurses, doctors, pastors, family and friends. Only the Lord knows how much we appreciate their goodness.

A special thanks also goes to Kathy Mahan, a registered nurse in our church. She and her husband Paul were some of our close friends. Kathy came almost every day for weeks and did things for Pam that I didn't have the medical knowledge to do. She brought her little boys with her, and my children took care of them while she worked with Pam. Kathy made a list of other nurses who were willing to help, and she coordinated the schedule. Nurses we had never met volunteered their help, along with those we did know: Ann Campbell, Mrs. Dale Ceren and others.

I also express my appreciation to the ladies who came and helped bathe Pam, do her hair, trim her nails, do the laundry and change her bed (as often as seven times a day).

Washing Pam's hair was quite an ordeal when we first took her home. She was still in a coma and was unable to help herself in any way. She had a tube in her nose and had to use a catheter. While I held Pam's head over a large garbage can, the ladies poured pans of water over her hair to wash and rinse it. How grateful we are for all of these friends!

I am very thankful, too, for Jim and Penne Rooney, the young couple from Miles City, Montana, working with us at that time. Penne and I took turns watching Pam through the vigil of Pam's early battle. She stayed with Pam for twelve hours, and I stayed twelve. The Rooneys also kept Pam while I went to Florida for Tim and Terry's wedding at Terry's home church. I was so happy for Tim and Terry; yet, it was so hard to stand in the receiving line, knowing that my precious wife, who had so diligently loved Tim and reared him as her own son, was not able to share in this blessed occasion.

A few days later we had a reception in Denver for Tim and Terry, and the church folks got to see Terry in her wedding gown. Pam was there, but she was still in a coma and did not comprehend what was happening.

In this chapter I would like to express appreciation to the assistant pastors at our church for their faithfulness to visit us. Brother Chuck Crabtree, one of the assistants, sang to Pam while she was in the coma, hoping that she would hear and be blessed. He and his wife Alyce are some of our very special friends.

I thank all you pastors who called, wrote, kept calling, kept writing and took special love offerings. Thank you!

For those pastors who took the time and money to fly to the hospital in Alexandria and be with us there, I give my special thanks. Many nights we saw as many as twenty-five men on their knees in the waiting room, crying out to God on behalf of my wife.

This chapter would not be complete without saying thank you to Mr. and Mrs. Warren Hosaflook for keeping our children while we were in Israel, and for opening their home to us during those early days of Pam's illness.

To family members from Texas who came to visit us in

the hospital in Denver and who faithfully called during the early weeks of our trial, I thank you.

To the Hlads and the Kriegers who came and sang to Pam while she was in the coma, I say thanks.

More precious than diamonds, silver, gold or all of this world's wealth are friends who pray, who give, who weep, who care. Thank God for friends!

CHAPTER 11

The Family

I close this book by letting you know some of the things that have taken place in the lives of various family members and the impact Pam's illness has had on them.

Pam's Family

Pam's mother and dad, Mr. and Mrs. Bill James, saw their daughter go from one of the smartest women they had ever known, to a total invalid. In the height of Pam's illness, they flew to Alexandria, Virginia, and spent a week with us. They came at other times and gave moral support. I thank God that Pam has a mother and dad who love the Lord Jesus Christ very dearly. They knew how to call upon Him for strength and have stayed close to the Lord through this trial. They have no bitterness in their hearts toward Him. They simply accept Pam's illness as the Lord's will for their lives and for ours.

I take this opportunity to say, "Thank you, Mom and Dad, for your sweet testimony, love and encouragement during these long months."

As I stated earlier, Pam's sister Peggy came back to the Lord through this trial and is living for Him. I'm sure that God used our situation to also speak to the hearts of Annette (Pam's youngest sister), her husband Larry and their precious children. I thank God for the encouraging letters that both Peggy and Annette wrote to us.

Our Children

Tim married in June after Pam became ill in March. He and Terry Griffin were already engaged, but he told me he was willing to wait about getting married until Pam got better. I felt they should go ahead with their plans, which they did.

Perhaps one of the hardest things was to perform the wedding ceremony and stand in the receiving line without my precious wife. She had become Tim's mother when Tim was three years of age and had so wonderfully raised him. She had waited for this hour, but she was still in a coma in Denver and was not even aware a wedding was taking place.

For the short while that Pam and Terry knew each other before Pam became ill, they shared some wonderful times. They talked, shopped and prayed together as though they had known each other for years. Pam was so excited about having Terry for a daughter-in-law. They enjoyed the same things and were so much alike. Many have commented that they even look alike and wondered if Terry were Pam's sister or daughter.

We thank God for our precious, sweet daughter-in-law and for the way she has so graciously carried the burden of our family. She has been a tremendous blessing to each of us and has expressed a great desire to help meet the needs of our family. Terry's testimony for the Lord is without spot, and her love for us has been overwhelming.

I'm so thankful that Tim didn't let Pam's illness make him bitter. The fact that God had taken his first mother, then struck down the one who had lovingly taken her place, could have been enough to stop him. But instead, he has gone on and preached to the glory of God.

Tim finished college and was in evangelism for a few years

before he began pastoring. He and Terry have three precious children—Chad, Tiffany and Troy.

Phyllis, our oldest daughter, was seventeen when Pam became ill. She had always been good to help Pam with the children and the housework, but she suddenly found herself thrust into a position of having to be the responsible person for seeing that these things were done all the time.

Pam and Phyllis had been close. As teenagers ought to, Phyllis would pour out her heart to her mother about the various bumps and lumps of her teenage years. Phyllis missed those times so very much. I'm sure she spent many moments of secret grieving over Pam's situation, though she never complained.

I tried to meet the needs of her heart, but no matter how much a daddy loves his daughter or how hard he tries to fill the gap, he can't take a mother's place.

In September after Pam became ill in March, Phyllis left for college. While she was at Bob Jones University, she would call and write to me, and I would call her and write to her. I flew down and took her shopping and tried to do what Pam would do if she were able, but I knew Phyllis's needs were not being met. But God gave her strength to carry on.

God was especially gracious when Phyllis came home for Christmas. Up to that time, Pam had not shown any emotion of any kind since she became ill. Before Phyllis got off the plane, I prayed, "Lord, it would sure be good if Pam could show some emotion toward Phyllis." And when she came down the ramp, Pam began to cry. Excitedly, she said, "There's Phyllis! There's Phyllis!"

Phyllis passed by us all and ran into the arms of her mother. What a time of weeping and rejoicing as Pam showed some emotion for the first time! I was glad that God allowed it to be just at the time when Phyllis so desperately needed it.

After Christmas, Phyllis went back to school and finished her freshman year. By the time she came home for the summer, Penny was beginning to cave in under the pressure of a twelve-year-old girl having to do so much of the cooking, laundry and housework. Phyllis relieved that pressure throughout the summer.

Then, when it was time to go back to school, Phyllis came to me and said, "Dad, I cannot return to college; I must stay home and help you and Penny take care of Mother."

I didn't want to ask Phyllis to give up her college career to help us, but we so desperately needed her at home. Even before Phyllis had told me she would not be returning to college, I had asked the Lord to touch her heart about it. I thank God for her sweet spirit and hard work.

The Lord blessed her unselfishness and later sent a young man into her life. She and Paul Williams (the same name as my second son) were married on May 29, 1981. They now have two sons, Christopher and Nicholas.

Our son Paul was fourteen when Pam became ill. In some ways this has been harder on him than on any of the others. Paul was at an age when he needed the understanding, sweetness and kindness of his mother's love.

I tried desperately to meet his needs. We had father-son talks, went hunting and did other things together; but I sensed he still had a void in his life that only his mother could fill.

Although, because of the intimacy, Paul couldn't help bathe or dress Pam, he did other things. He vacuumed, helped around the house and was willing to do for his mother everything that he could do. He stayed with her many times, went to get things she needed and was very loving toward her.

It still thrills my heart to think of the many times he would come to our bedroom, put his arms around his mother and kiss her goodnight.

Paul is still very affectionate to his mother, and they enjoy spending time together. I thank God for his kind, sweet attitude toward her.

Paul married Jeanne Ohler in August, 1984, and God

blessed them with two precious children—Pamela Jeanne (born on Paul's birthday on May 4, 1986) and Thomas Paul II (born April 21, 1987).

Penny turned eleven on March 10—the very next day after Pam went into a coma. Pam had always made birthdays a special time, so it was especially heartbreaking for her to be ill for this occasion in Penny's life.

I was so pleased when the folks at Fairfax Baptist Temple organized a birthday party for Penny. They probably didn't realize what a tremendous need they were meeting in Penny's life and in ours by their gesture of kindness.

Penny carried a tremendous load of responsibility, especially after Phyllis left for college. I thank the Lord for her love and care for her mother. God only knows how many times Penny bathed her mother, shampooed her hair and fixed it the best she could at her young age. She diligently made the beds and did the laundry, sometimes staying up late at night to finish the work. Along with the work, she kept up with her schooling. This was hard on her, but she did not complain or question why God sent this trial to our family.

I say to her in this book what I have said to her so often, "Penny, I am so proud of you!"

Like Pam, Penny married when she was only seventeen. She and her husband, Todd Lehigh, live in Montana.

The Scriptures say that children are a "heritage of the Lord" (Ps. 127:3). Our children surely have made the difference in our trial. I have no idea how I could have managed without them.

Many people have come to me down through the years and said, "Brother Williams, you have some of the sweetest daughters in the world. They care for their mother so wonderfully."

How good and precious they have been! Only Heaven will record the countless number of times I have bowed my head and thanked God for my children. They have filled a space in my life that could not be filled by anything else. Thank you, Tim, Phyllis, Paul and Penny. I owe you so much.

My Situation

Let me say that I, as Pam's husband, have been thankful to God for this opportunity to demonstrate my love for my wife. Many pastors and others have said, "Tom, thank you for your testimony of being faithful to Pam, for caring and loving and demonstrating what a husband really ought to be."

Actually, it has been my privilege to care for her, to give myself for her as Christ gave Himself for the church. You see, when she was able, Pam was the finest, most precious wife that a man could possibly have. She was a wonderful mother, a gourmet cook and a tremendous hostess, entertaining more than five hundred people a year in our home.

Pam did all of my secretarial work. She could type one hundred words a minute and take dictation as fast as I could give it. She was always thinking of ways to help me.

I have no bitterness in my heart toward the Lord—only love and gratitude that He trusted our family with this trial. I can say honestly that I love the Lord more now than ever before. I probably appreciate my wife and children more than most because I have been taught to do so by this event.

We have not been bankrupted as a family by Pam's illness; instead, our relationship has been made very, very rich. We thank God for His love and mercy during our trial—not only the past few years, but still today as I, along with her full-time nurse, continue working with Pam.